# HIPAA
## Handbook
# for Business Associates

Understanding the Privacy
and Security Regulations

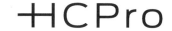

*HIPAA Handbook for Business Associates: Understanding the Privacy and Security Regulations* is published by HCPro, Inc.

ISBN: 978-1-61569-225-5

HCPro, Inc., provides information resources for the healthcare industry. HCPro, Inc., is not affiliated in any way with The Joint Commission, which owns the JCAHO and Joint Commission trademarks.

Kate Borten, CISSP, CISM, Author
Gerianne Spanek, Managing Editor
Mary Stevens, Editor
James T. DeWolf, Publisher and Editorial Director
Mike Mirabello, Production Specialist
Amanda Donaldson, Proofreader
Matt Sharpe, Senior Manager of Production
Shane Katz, Art Director
Jean St. Pierre, Vice President of Operations and Customer Service

Advice given is general. Readers should consult professional counsel for specific legal, ethical, or clinical questions. Arrangements can be made for quantity discounts. For more information, contact:

HCPro, Inc.
75 Sylvan Street, Suite A-101
Danvers, MA 01923
Telephone: 800-650-6787 or 781-639-1872
Fax: 800-639-8511
Email: *customerservice@hcpro.com*

**Visit HCPro online at: *www.hcpro.com* and *www.hcmarketplace.com*.**

05/2013
22032

# CONTENTS

# ABOUT THE AUTHOR

## Kate Borten, CISSP, CISM

Kate Borten, president of The Marblehead Group, offers a unique blend of technical and management expertise, information security and privacy knowledge, and an insider's understanding of the healthcare industry. Her company, founded in 1999, serves the full spectrum of covered entities and their business associates with respect to understanding privacy and security regulations, establishing and enhancing their formal privacy and security programs, and assessing risk and regulatory compliance.

Borten has more than 20 years of experience designing, implementing, and integrating healthcare information systems at world-renowned medical facilities, including Massachusetts General Hospital, where she was responsible for system development. Before founding The Marblehead Group, Borten served as chief information security officer at CareGroup, Inc., where she established a comprehensive information security program that encompassed all entities within this major Boston-area integrated healthcare delivery system. She is an internationally certified information security professional, an Information Systems Security Association (ISSA™) senior member, and a member of the New England chapter's board of directors. She has chaired health sector information security and privacy national conferences and frequently speaks on these topics.

# HIPAA Handbook
## for Business Associates
*Understanding the Privacy and Security Regulations*

## Intended Audience

You work for an organization that is designated as a business associate (BA) of one or more Health Insurance Portability and Accountability Act of 1996 (HIPAA) covered entities (CE) or of another BA. This means your organization provides some service for or on behalf of a healthcare provider or payer, directly or indirectly, and that service involves access to protected health information.

Many kinds of organizations can be designated as BAs, including the following:

- Certain consulting firms

- Coding and billing services

- Transcription services

- Collection agencies

- Record/data storage and disposal companies

- Certain attorneys and auditors

- Professional management services

- Electronic health record vendors

- Certain personal health record vendors

- Information technology (IT) management and support companies, including cloud vendors

- Health information organizations and regional health networks

- E-prescribing gateways

- Patient safety organizations

- Accreditation agencies

## Learning Objectives

After reading this handbook, you should be able to do the following:

- Understand what HIPAA and the Healthcare Information Technology for Economic and Clinical Health (HITECH) Act are and how they affect BAs and their workforce

- Understand what constitutes protected health information

- Protect patient privacy while performing BA-related tasks

- Recognize the permissible uses and disclosures of protected health information

- Identify safe ways to handle email and faxes containing PHI

- Protect protected health information both inside the organization and off-site

- Create effective passwords to protect electronic information

## HIPAA, the HITECH Act, and Omnibus Rule Overview

HIPAA requires privacy and security protections for individually identifiable patient and health plan member information or protected health information. The HIPAA Privacy and Security Rules require CEs to have special contracts with their BAs to pass on many of these obligations, making BAs contractually liable.

The American Recovery and Reinvestment Act of 2009 includes a subset called the HITECH Act, which, extends direct liability to BAs for compliance with HIPAA's Security Rule and certain portions of HIPAA's Privacy and Breach Notification Rules. Until enactment of the HITECH Act, the U.S. Department of Health and Human Services (HHS) could enforce only CEs' compliance with HIPAA rules. Now BAs have both direct liability to the federal government and contractual liability to the CE with which it signed a BA contract.

The 2013 Modifications to the HIPAA Privacy, Security, Enforcement, and Breach Notification Rules under the Health Information

Technology for Economic and Clinical Health Act and the Genetic Information Nondiscrimination Act (Omnibus Rule) makes BAs directly liable for the following:

- Failure to comply with the HIPAA Security Rule

- Uses and disclosures of protected health information that are impermissible according to the HIPAA Privacy Rule

- Failure to provide access to electronic protected health information when requested by the individual who is the subject of the protected health information, or by the relevant CE on behalf of the individual

- Failure to provide an accounting of certain protected health information disclosures as required by the Privacy Rule

- Failure to provide breach notification as required by the Breach Notification Rule

- Failure to provide protected health information to HHS when required by an investigation or to determine the BA's compliance

The HITECH Act further includes provisions for heightened enforcement of HIPAA and stiffer penalties for noncompliance and privacy and security violations. It also is the first federal law to require notification in case of a breach of a patient's or plan member's information.

The 2013 Omnibus Rule implements many of the HITECH Act requirements and goes further. Directly relevant to BAs, the Omnibus

Rule expands the definition of a BA to include all of a BA's downstream subcontractors with access to protected health information. BAs generally are required to pass along the same contractual obligations and limits to its downstream subcontractors that it has to its upstream BAs or CEs. Note that the Omnibus Rule revises some required language in BA contracts.

Your organization must ensure that HIPAA-compliant BA contracts are signed before permitting another person or entity to have access to protected health information for which you are responsible. Contracts must specify that subcontractors will do the same if they subcontract. If a subcontractor discovers a privacy or security incident or breach, the incident must be reported up the chain to the affected CEs.

### HIPAA and you

As a BA, you might have access to protected health information, you might have a business need to discuss protected health information with colleagues and third parties, and you might communicate with patients or health plan members and even members of their families. The HITECH Act and Omnibus Rule changes make understanding HIPAA privacy and security requirements particularly important.

## Terms You Should Know

### Protected health information or PHI

HIPAA and your organization's BA contracts establish rules for when and how protected health information or PHI may be used and released. So it is essential to understand what constitutes PHI.

PHI includes any information that can be linked to a specific patient or health plan member. PHI can take any form. It can be electronic, written, or spoken.

PHI may include obvious identifiers such as name, medical record number, or insurance subscriber number. However, information without obvious identifiers can still point to one individual. For example, if only one patient underwent a particular medical procedure this week, the procedure would be enough to identify that patient and would be PHI. Alternatively, if only one health plan member is a goat herder residing in New York City, this occupation combined with residence would be enough to identify this individual.

PHI includes demographic information about a patient, as well as financial and health information if it can be linked to a specific patient. PHI includes billing and insurance claims information, insurance eligibility and coverage, the reason a person is sick or in the hospital, treatments and medications a patient may receive, test results, photographs and radiology images, allergies, observations about a patient's condition, information about past health conditions or treatments, discharge planning information, and more. The Omnibus Rule explicitly adds genetic information about individuals and their family members to the definition of PHI.

### Minimum necessary/need to know

HIPAA requires that BAs follow the principle of minimum necessary when using, disclosing, and requesting PHI. Otherwise, it is an impermissible use, disclosure, or request under the Privacy Rule.

Only individuals with an authorized "need to know" to perform their jobs may have access to PHI. Furthermore, individuals with access to PHI may access and release only the minimum necessary PHI to perform their jobs.

Your use and disclosure of PHI must also comply with your organization's BA contracts. BA contracts specify which functions or services your organization is performing that put your organization in contact with PHI. Other than performing these functions or services, there are limited other purposes for which your organization is permitted to use or disclose PHI. You must ensure that you access and release PHI only as permitted by your organization's contracts and policies.

Ask yourself the following questions before you access any patient information:

- Do I need this information to perform my job?

- What is the least amount of information I need to perform my job?

- To whom am I releasing the information, and is that person or entity permitted to have it?

- Does this use or disclosure comply with HIPAA and our BA contracts?

Ensure that you release only the minimum necessary PHI in response to a request or to serve a particular purpose. When you release PHI, even if another party has requested more PHI, your organization is responsible if the PHI is excessive. Violation of the minimum necessary principle is a HIPAA violation and can result in federal penalties for BAs. If you are unsure about a certain situation, consult your privacy officer, compliance officer, or information security officer (ISO).

## Case scenario #1: Celebrity sighting

You work for a billing company and you are preparing a patient bill when you recognize the patient's name—he's the shortstop for the Chicago Cubs. Apparently, physicians at the hospital for which your company provides billing services performed an outpatient procedure on his shoulder.

During a break later in the day, you call a friend who works at the hospital to learn more about the famous patient. She cared for the patient and discusses his condition. You chat for a few more minutes, but you think about the conversation as you prepare to return to work.

The conversation was not malicious, and it was between friends, so it seems harmless. But something tells you it was inappropriate.

 **Did you do anything wrong?**

 Yes. You and your friend violated HIPAA, and this was potentially a breach. You must report it to your supervisor, privacy officer, or other designated leader for investigation. You regret that it happened and you realize that you had no business inquiring about the patient because it had nothing to do with your job. Your friend made matters worse because she should not have told you that she cared for this celebrity or discussed him with you. This is a HIPAA privacy violation, despite your belief that the conversation was harmless.

Patients' right to privacy has been violated in some well-publicized cases, such as when actor George Clooney received treatment after a motorcycle accident and when former President Bill Clinton underwent cardiac surgery. In both cases, staff members and physicians accessed the patient's information strictly out of curiosity, not for a work-related need. Disciplinary action ensued, and the facilities involved endured public embarrassment.

## Privacy Rights of Patients and Health Plan Members

BAs are both directly liable and contractually liable for supporting certain privacy rights of individuals.

### Access to one's PHI

Patients and plan members generally have a right to view and receive a copy of their PHI in a designated record set. Each BA and CE or upstream BA must agree contractually whether the BA has PHI in a designated record set as determined by the original CE and, if so, how and by whom requests for access and copies will be handled. The Omnibus Rule strengthens individuals' right to receive electronic copies when PHI is in electronic form, and the right to have their PHI transmitted, in any form, to a third party.

### Amending PHI

Patients and plan members have a right to request amendments to their PHI. Unlike updating an address or insurance plan, this refers to amending substantive information, particularly when relevant to a patient's care. For example, a patient may view his or her medical record and notice that a laboratory test is missing or incomplete. The patient may then request that an amendment be added to the record. CEs are not required to agree, but if they do, the PHI held by BAs may require amendment. BAs and CEs should agree on procedures for this situation.

## Restrictions on PHI use and disclosure

Patients and plan members have a right to request restrictions on how their PHI is used and disclosed or to whom. Generally, CEs are not required to agree. However, the Omnibus Rule requires healthcare providers to agree when a patient requests that a claim not be submitted for a service or item for which the patient pays in full out of pocket. Any restriction that a CE agrees to must be strictly upheld. Some restrictions may affect BAs; they and CEs should agree on how to respond when this occurs.

## Accounting of disclosures

Patients and plan members have a right to request and receive an accounting of certain PHI disclosures occurring during the previous six years. This accounting or report excludes disclosures for treatment, payment, healthcare operations, and disclosures the patient or plan member has authorized. Many possible disclosures must be tracked (e.g., disclosures made for public health purposes). BAs are directly responsible for knowing which disclosures require tracking and, if relevant to the BA's circumstances, tracking all such disclosures. Furthermore, BAs must have an on-demand retrieval and reporting process to respond within 60 days of an individual's accounting request.

### Confidential communications

Patients and plan members have a right to request that they be contacted via alternative means to ensure confidentiality. This is typically an alternative telephone number or mailing address, such as a post office box. When CEs agree (healthcare providers are required to agree), it must be strictly upheld. Agreements to alternative communications are likely to affect BAs with patient and plan member contact. Therefore, CEs and BAs should agree on how to communicate and implement such agreements.

If you are involved in any of these activities, ensure that you know and comply with your organization's policies and procedures before releasing any PHI.

## Privacy in Your Organization

Patients receiving healthcare expect privacy whether they are in a hospital, physician's office, laboratory, or other healthcare setting. Health plan members also expect privacy regarding their health status and services received. Even though your job may only indirectly involve patient care or payment for services, you still play a role in protecting individuals' privacy. You should use or disclose PHI only when necessary to perform your job.

### How you can protect individuals' privacy

The following measures can help you keep PHI confidential:

- Ensure that paper documents and records with PHI are in locked storage, and allow access only to those individuals who need this information to perform their jobs.

- If you use electronic records, always log off your computer when you leave your desk, and never leave your laptop computer, tablet, or smartphone connected and unattended.

- Turn computer screens away from the view of the public or others with no need to know, or use privacy filters to ensure that unauthorized individuals don't view the information inadvertently.

- Cross-shred any CDs and paper that contain PHI before discarding them or place them in designated locked bins for secure disposal.

### High-risk situations: Faxing

HIPAA protects faxed PHI. Remember that faxed patient and plan member information can easily fall into the wrong hands. This would be a privacy violation. Faxing is a risky way to transmit PHI for two reasons:

1. You might dial the fax number incorrectly

2. Recipients might have changed the fax numbers that you have filed or programmed into your computer or fax machine

Before faxing any PHI, ensure that you know and follow your company's fax policy and procedures and any limits on its use. Use the following tips to avoid unauthorized disclosure of PHI via fax:

- Use a cover page that includes a confidentiality message

- Verify the intended recipient's fax number and ensure that you are sending the fax to the correct person at the correct number

- Confirm with the recipient that you are sending the information to a dedicated fax machine in a secure location

- Ensure that the recipient of the faxed information is authorized to receive it

- Call to confirm that this individual actually received the fax

- Ask individuals who send you faxes to notify you beforehand so you can be present to retrieve them immediately upon receipt

- Retrieve documents from your fax machine immediately upon receipt

## High-risk situations: Email

Sending email containing PHI outside your organization is very risky. Messages can easily be intercepted via the Internet. Using encrypted email is the best protection. Some organizations prohibit sending email containing PHI outside the organization. Ensure that you know and follow your organization's rules.

Confirm that you are sending your email to the correct recipient. This is a sound business practice, because sending unencrypted email containing patient or plan member information to the wrong individual is presumed to be a breach under the rules. If you are permitted to send PHI in unencrypted email, be discreet and avoid including patient and plan member names if possible.

## High-risk situations: Printed PHI

Don't leave documents containing PHI strewn about. The wrong person, including cleaning or maintenance staff members, can retrieve printouts, copies of records, or casual notes left on copiers, printers, fax machines, and desks.

Never take PHI outside your facility unless organization policy permits it and your supervisor grants specific permission for you to do so.

## High-risk situations: Working off-site

Working off-site creates potential privacy and security risks. Don't work off-site unless you have your organization's approval, and then be sure to follow your organization's policy and rules.

If you work off-site, use the following tips to help protect PHI:

- Transport portable devices and media (electronic and paper) in locked cases

- Password-protect devices and encrypt data

- Shred paper and CDs when no longer needed

- Never leave your desktop or laptop computer, tablet, or smartphone logged on and unattended if the device contains or accesses PHI

- Be especially aware of who can see your computer screen and overhear confidential conversations

# Security

Privacy and security are directly related. Many of the security measures discussed here are used to protect privacy and confidentiality.

The HITECH Act and Omnibus Rule require that all BAs comply fully with the HIPAA Security Rule. HIPAA's security requirements are designed to safeguard electronic PHI. However, the Privacy Rule requires security safeguards for all forms of PHI. Your organization is required to implement a comprehensive information security program, including administrative, physical, and technical measures. In addition to written policies and procedures, your organization is responsible for ongoing security awareness and training of its workforce. Distributing this handbook is one way your organization complies.

Security requirements apply to all PHI everywhere, including data stored on hard drives, removable and portable memory devices (e.g., laptop computers and USB thumb drives), and data sent via the Internet or included in email.

## Security: What you can do

Your organization is required to appoint an information security officer (ISO) with responsibility for the program. Ensure that you know who this is and how to contact this individual. Despite having an ISO, the administrative, physical, and technical safeguards intended to secure PHI in your organization are insufficient unless everyone cooperates.

You can contribute to information security by doing the following:

- Properly managing your password

- Preventing the spread of viruses

- Logging off your computer

- Being aware of and responsible for any PHI taken or accessed off-site

## Security: What your organization must do

Your organization should use these measures to safeguard PHI:

- Monitor login attempts

- Respond to information security incidents

- Protect computers from viruses and malicious software

- Protect patient or plan member information that is removed from the facility or accessed from off-site locations

- Educate employees and other workforce members about your written security policies and procedures, as well as security risks and countermeasures

- Educate the workforce about the consequences of violating policies and procedures, including disciplinary and legal action

## Examples of safeguards

Examples of safeguards that your company must establish include the following:

- **Administrative safeguards** such as security policies and training, risk assessments and risk management, compliance reviews, a sanctions policy, setup and termination-of-access procedures, incident and breach response, data backup and disaster recovery plans, and subcontractor BA contracts

- **Physical safeguards** such as locks and building security systems, workstation and portable device/media controls, and processes for secure erasure and disposal of PHI (preferably meeting National Institute of Standards and Technology guidelines)

- **Technical safeguards** such as unique user IDs, adequate user authentication, automatic inactivity logoff of systems with PHI, capture and review of audit logs, encryption of PHI at rest and in transit when warranted by risk, and data integrity controls

## Ways to ensure physical security

Information security relies on technical measures such as passwords, but physical security also plays an important role. The following measures can help ensure physical security:

- Ensure that your computer screen cannot be seen from public areas, or use a privacy filter.

- Lock laptop computers and other portable devices when not in use.

- Secure disks, CDs, USB drives, and other storage devices containing PHI in locked containers or cabinets.

- Follow your organization's policies for turning off or logging off your computer when you leave your desk.

- Use password-protected screensavers or keyboard-locking capabilities that your organization has made available. Don't attempt to disable these features if they are installed on your computer.

- Practice commonsense security. Lock doors and desks if appropriate to do so.

- Adhere to a clean desk policy and secure all confidential papers and electronic media in a locked container or cabinet before leaving your area.

- Shred all paper and CDs containing confidential information, including PHI, before discarding them or store them in designated locked bins for secure disposal.

## Paper record storage

BAs must exercise care when storing any paper records that contain PHI. The size of your organization and the physical layout of your facility will determine your optimum storage methods.

Do your part to keep your records safe. If your organization stores inactive or archived paper records on-site, close and lock the door to the storage space to prevent unauthorized access. Access records only when necessary to perform your job.

## Personal user IDs and passwords

HIPAA requires that individuals have and use their own unique user IDs. This allows organizations to know who views and updates which information. Anyone with access to PHI must have a unique user ID (login ID or login name), so computer systems can track every user's activity. This is standard security practice and should be company policy.

Never allow anyone to use your ID and password to log in to the computer system. Also never log in for someone else, even if you know the person has a work-related need. These are security violations, and you will be responsible for the other individual's computer activity. Similarly, don't ask others for permission to use their IDs and passwords.

Selecting a strong password—one that others can't guess easily—is an essential step in securing your organization's information. Generally, you should use a password that does the following:

- Includes both letters and numbers

- Isn't a personal name, special date, fictional character, or real word

- Consists of at least seven or eight characters

- Incorporates both upper- and lowercase letters

- Incorporates special keyboard characters (e.g., #, !, or $) if your system can support them

- Is difficult for others to guess but easy for you to remember

Change your password regularly. Doing so at least once every three months is a good rule of thumb. Be sure to change your password if you think someone else knows it. Follow your organization's policy.

### Case scenario #2: Pass on the weak password

Jennifer Jones, a consultant who performs medical record reviews for CEs, has not changed her computer password in several months and thinks it is time to do so. She is fairly certain that she can think of something better than her current password, "jjones," and she wants to make her new password as secure as possible.

 **Which of the following is her best choice?**

- **JjOnEs—She added some odd capitalization**

- **JJ!Atlan98—She combined numbers, letters, the year she moved to Atlanta, and a special character**

- **jj0ne5—She changed the O to a zero, and the S to a five**

- **JenJ—She used a different variation of her name that is different but still easy for her to remember**

**A** JJ!Atlan98 is the best password option. It combines numbers, upper- and lowercase letters, and a special character (the exclamation point), and it is not based solely on her name. It's a good thing she's changing it because her previous password is very weak and easy to guess.

## Protecting against computer viruses

A computer virus or other malicious software can destroy information stored on your computer. It also can copy your passwords or PHI that you store or send. Viruses often are transmitted via email attachments or by visiting certain websites.

## Unauthorized software

Music-sharing and remote access software, games, and other programs that you may want to install can disable your computer, threaten your organization's network, and contain malicious software that would allow hackers to access your computer. Don't install any software on your computer without permission from your IT department.

Make special note of file types before opening them. Files that end with ".exe" are executable files, or software programs. Viruses or malicious software programs often are contained in downloaded executable files. Do not open these files without permission from your technical support department.

## DOS AND DON'TS FOR PROTECTING AGAINST VIRUSES

| Dos | Don'ts |
|---|---|
| Do tell your IT department if you receive an unrecognizable or suspicious email or if an unfamiliar program appears on your computer. | Don't open suspicious email and attachments from unrecognized senders. |
| Do follow your organization's policy for using antivirus software and keep it up to date. | Don't uninstall or disable any antivirus applications installed on your computer. |
| Do use your email in a manner that is consistent with your facility's policies and procedures. | Never forward work email to your personal account (e.g., Hotmail® or Gmail™). Don't access personal email accounts while you are at work unless permitted to do so. |

### *Case scenario #3: Installing software*

You want to install iTunes® on your work computer so you can charge your iPod® for the long drive home.

 **What should you do?**

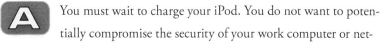 You must wait to charge your iPod. You do not want to potentially compromise the security of your work computer or network. Be sure to follow your organization's policy on downloading software.

## Unauthorized hardware

Exercise similar precautions when installing hardware. Any device attached to your organization's network or your computer must be installed with the appropriate security precautions in mind.

This is why you should connect devices such as computers and servers to the network only if you have permission to do so from your technical support staff. The same rule applies for connecting devices to your computer—via the USB port, for example.

Some organizations prohibit the use of personally owned computers—including desktop and laptop computers, tablets, and smartphones—for work. Other organizations permit these user-owned devices but require that the operating system, antivirus software, Web browser, and other components remain up to date. Ensure that you know and follow your organization's requirements.

## Email security

Information that you send via email generally is not secure. This is why BAs should adopt strict policies that govern how they transmit PHI electronically. Your organization's email program may encrypt the information before sending it, or you may have special Web-based tools for securely transmitting PHI. Some organizations ban inclusion of PHI in email. Ensure that you know and follow your organization's email policy.

## *Encryption*

Encryption simply means that information is coded or scrambled so that anyone who lacks the key to read it cannot do so. Many BAs encrypt confidential data they store or transmit depending on the level of risk that an unauthorized individual might read it. Many state breach notification laws and the HIPAA Breach Notification Rule consider properly encrypted data to be safe from disclosure and breach.

PHI is at a higher-than-average security risk if it is:

- Transmitted via the Internet or a wireless network

- Stored on portable devices (e.g., laptop computers, tablets, and smartphones such as an iPhone™ or BlackBerry®)

- Stored on portable media (e.g., disks and USB drives)

Many companies now require encryption in these situations. Often, software programs that encrypt data operate invisibly to users. You must know whether your organization requires that you take steps to encrypt data.

## *Protecting laptop computers and other portable devices*

Many individuals use portable computers, including laptop computers, tablets, and smartphones for work. The most frequent associated risks of doing so are loss or theft of these devices. Loss of equipment and potential loss of data confidentiality are the unfortunate result. If your device or portable media (e.g., CD or USB thumb drive) with PHI is lost or stolen, you must file an incident report with your facility immediately.

Use the following tips to protect laptop computers and other portable devices and media:

- Don't save PHI on portable devices and media unless they're protected by a password and encryption

- Don't store passwords and access codes on your portable device

- Back up information stored on your portable device if it is unique source data

- Pay special attention to portable media (e.g., disks, CDs, or USB thumb drives) that you take off-site

- Lock portable devices and media in a secure container, cabinet, or briefcase when not in use

## Case scenario #4: The cost of buying gas suddenly went way, way up

You work for an auditing company that serves as a BA to many CEs. You are able to work from home two days a week. Your company has issued you a laptop computer for this purpose and you take special precautions—you don't allow your children to use it, you update your antivirus software, and you use a strong password when you log in. However, one program you use is not working, so you bring the laptop computer the next time you go to your office.

Your technical support department returns the laptop computer to you in great condition. You take it with you when you leave the office. En route home, you stop to purchase gas. Without thinking about it, you leave the laptop computer and your other belongings on the front passenger seat while you pump the gas and go inside to pay for it.

Upon arriving home, you realize that your laptop computer is missing. You recall that you left your car unlocked and your window halfway down while you were at the gas station. Apparently, while you were inside, someone else left the station with a full tank—and a new laptop computer containing more patient information than you care to acknowledge.

 **What should you do?**

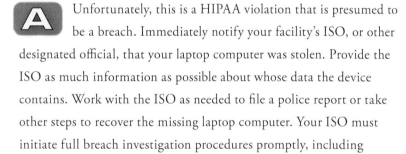 Unfortunately, this is a HIPAA violation that is presumed to be a breach. Immediately notify your facility's ISO, or other designated official, that your laptop computer was stolen. Provide the ISO as much information as possible about whose data the device contains. Work with the ISO as needed to file a police report or take other steps to recover the missing laptop computer. Your ISO must initiate full breach investigation procedures promptly, including preparing to notify affected CEs or upstream BAs.

You know that you should not have left the laptop computer unattended and in view in your unlocked vehicle. You should have taken it with you into the gas station or hidden it and locked the car. At least if the PHI had been encrypted, the loss would be limited to the value of the laptop computer and lost time and aggravation. Take every possible precaution with portable media—keep them in sight, password-protect devices, and encrypt confidential information. Review your company's policy pertaining to laptop computer and portable device security for other precautions and safeguards you should take.

## The Consequences of Breaking the Rules

HIPAA's Security Rule requires BAs to implement a sanctions policy to address situations involving employees and other workforce members who violate HIPAA privacy and security regulations and organization policy. In addition to internal sanctions, there may be severe external consequences.

Violating HIPAA's Privacy, Security, or Breach Notification Rules can result in civil or criminal penalties. The civil penalties finalized by the Omnibus Rule are based on a four-tier system of increasing penalties, depending on factors such as willful neglect. Civil penalties include fines of up to $1.5 million for repeated violations of a single requirement in a calendar year.

Criminal penalties for wrongful disclosure of patient information can include large fines and incarceration for up to 10 years. Wrongful disclosure includes obtaining PHI with the intent to sell, transfer, or use it for personal gain, commercial advantage, or malicious harm.

### *Reporting violations*

Your organization expects all employees and other workforce members to adhere to its privacy and security policies, but it recognizes that some people may break the rules. Under HIPAA, your organization's responsibilities include monitoring compliance and investigating any privacy/security complaints, violations, and breaches.

You must report all violations and suspected violations immediately to your facility's privacy official or information security official or as instructed by your facility's procedures. Your organization may also provide a way for you to report them anonymously, such as via a telephone compliance hotline. Do not fear retaliation if you report a violation. Your organization may not punish employees for reporting violations. Your responsibilities include reporting instances in which you suspect that someone is violating the privacy or security policies.

### *If your facility experiences a breach*

Your facility is required to implement procedures for responding to a privacy or security problem involving PHI, and you should know beforehand what your role is, if any, in these procedures.

The HITECH Act defines breach as any unauthorized access, acquisition, use, or disclosure of PHI that compromises the privacy or security of this information. Under the 2013 Omnibus Rule, privacy and security violations involving PHI are presumed to be breaches, with several important exceptions. Organizations are required to have documented procedures to make this determination and to respond as required by the Breach Notification Rule.

Under the Breach Notification Rule, when a breach affecting PHI under the control of a BA occurs, the BA must notify the affected CEs or upstream BAs no later than 60 days from discovery. A breach is considered discovered on the first day a person or organization knows or should have known about it.

However, BA contracts almost always require that BAs notify the upstream partner rapidly (e.g., within several business days) of any privacy or security incident or violation involving PHI. It is important, and required, for every employee and workforce member to report even a suspected privacy or security violation or breach as soon as they are aware of it, because the clock is ticking.

CEs are responsible for providing breach notification to affected patients or plan members and to HHS. However, based on contractual agreements and other factors, your organization may be required to provide notification. BAs should ensure that their privacy and security incident response plan and procedures are sufficiently detailed to address this possibility.

## Obtaining Help

You may have questions about HIPAA compliance or other compliance matters at your facility. Privacy and security are sometimes complex, so don't hesitate to contact your privacy officer, ISO, or other designated leader with questions. These individuals will be glad to assist you.

## In Conclusion

Complying with HIPAA is more important than ever for BAs. Pursuant to the HITECH Act, BAs now must comply with HIPAA's Security Rule and portions of its Privacy Rule. They are also subject to the same enforcement as CEs.

Having the right policies and security software is not sufficient. Each employee and workforce member must adhere to these policies and take an active role in your company's compliance efforts.

As you perform your job, remember the importance of the privacy and security of the patient and plan member data that you may encounter. Focusing on these essentials will help you ensure that your company is in compliance with HIPAA and the HITECH Act.

# FINAL EXAM

1.  **Your administrative assistant, Elizabeth, just began working at your consulting firm. You are conducting data analysis for a CE. You need her to retrieve some of your data tables that contain PHI. However, Elizabeth hasn't yet received her user ID (login name). What should you do?**

    a.  Let Elizabeth use your login name and password just this once; then change your password afterward

    b.  Darren, your former assistant, left last week; his login name and password, which he kept under his mousepad, are probably still active, so give Elizabeth this information

    c.  Log in with your own login name and password and let Elizabeth use your account for a few minutes

    d.  Contact your technical support department and ask whether it can create Elizabeth's login name and password quickly

2.  **Which of the following passwords is most secure?**

    a.  TMObg!31

    b.  BaseBALL

    c.  DavidOrtiz

    d.  2013RedSox

3. You're home at night relaxing and spending time on your personal computer. You check on your friend from the office. She posted a blog about her horrible day, describing her late arrival due to heavy traffic and the difficult claims she was responsible for billing that day. Unfortunately, she went into great detail. She even included descriptions of the unusual medical conditions of several patients whose claims she was completing. However, she didn't include the patients' names. What should you do?

   a. Email your coworker and tell her that she should consider making her blog private, just in case.

   b. Email your coworker and tell her that she should consider deleting the blog to be safe.

   c. Speak with your company's privacy or information security officer to determine whether this is a problem.

   d. Nothing. Let your friend vent. You shouldn't betray your coworker; she carefully avoided using patient names.

4. You conduct medical record reviews and your company allows you to work remotely. You are at home when you need to email a physician advisor some codes for review. However, your work email account unexpectedly is not functioning. What should you do?

   a. Use your personal email account to send the file

   b. Wait until your work email account is functioning again to send the codes

   c. Access the Internet via your cell phone and use it to send the email to the physician advisor

   d. Ask the physician advisor to download an instant messaging program, and send the file via that program

5. **Whom should you call if you suspect that another employee has violated HIPAA?**

   a. *60 Minutes*

   b. Your company's privacy or information security officer

   c. The police department

   d. Another employee to obtain his or her opinion

6. **Which of these practices does not ensure security?**

   a. Turning your computer screen away from public areas

   b. Locking laptop computers and other portable devices in secure containers or cabinets when not in use

   c. Leaving a shared computer on so your coworker doesn't have to log in again

   d. Ensuring that doors and desks are locked appropriately

7. **Which of the following practices does not protect against malicious software?**

   a. Avoiding opening unknown email attachments or email from unrecognized senders

   b. Ensuring that your computer antivirus software is up to date

   c. Downloading files from unfamiliar websites

   d. Scanning files that you created on another computer for viruses

8. **Which of these is a good security practice when you use a laptop computer or other portable device?**

   a. Saving PHI on the device without requiring a password

   b. Saving passwords and access codes on your device

   c. Updating your antivirus software

   d. Disabling encryption on the device

9. **Under which circumstances may you disclose PHI that you access on the job?**

   a. After you no longer work for the company

   b. When you think no one will be able to identify the patient

   c. If you think the patient won't mind

   d. When your job requires you to do so

10. **Your friend's father just underwent triple bypass surgery at one of the facilities for which you provide transcription services. Your friend asks if you can obtain information about his prognosis. What should you do?**

    a. Call a nurse you know who works at the hospital, and inquire about the patient's condition

    b. Log in to the computerized transcription system so you can read the patient's record to find this information for your friend

    c. Explain to your friend that viewing the patient's record or asking others for this information violates patient privacy and HIPAA

    d. Relay the information to your friend when you transcribe documentation from her father's surgery

# ANSWER KEY

| | | | |
|---|---|---|---|
| 1. | d | 6. | c |
| 2. | a | 7. | c |
| 3. | c | 8. | c |
| 4. | b | 9. | d |
| 5. | b | 10. | c |

# CERTIFICATE OF COMPLETION

This is to certify that

has read and successfully passed the final exam of

*HIPAA Handbook for Business Associates:*
*Understanding the Privacy and Security Regulations*

Geri Spanek, Managing Editor